Time To Stop Dieting and Start Living

Simple Ways to Start Enjoying Your Health

ADAM BORDES

AmErica House
Baltimore

ISBN: 1–58851–149–9
PUBLISHED BY AMERICA HOUSE
BOOK PUBLISHERS
www.publishamerica.com
Baltimore

Printed in the United States of America

DEDICATION

I would like to thank all of the amazing people who have touched my life in such a profound way. First and foremost, I would like to thank my family whose love and encouragement has inspired me to always be the best that I can be. To all of my instructors at The Florida State University who have taught me, as well as those I continue to learn from every single day at Logan College of Chiropractic, I am forever grateful for all of your wisdom. I would also like to thank all of my friends who have kept me sane from the beginning, thanks guys!

This book is being dedicated to those whose lives were forever changed on September 11, 2001. This day will live in infamy as it has united us as a nation and unleashed a passion within those of us who are proud to call The United States of America our home. To all of the brave individuals who gave their lives to serve others, these are the true heroes. May we all be so fortunate as to live our lives in service of our fellow man...

TABLE OF CONTENTS

The Fitness Revolution

PART I
Getting Started on Changing Your Life

PART II
Weight Loss and Weight Control

PART III
Becoming an Educated
Health and Fitness Consumer

PART IV

Beginning Your Fitness
and Exercise Program

PART V

The Future of Your Health

The Fitness Revolution

The dawn of a new era is upon us. With this new millennium bears with it the responsibility of people from all walks of life, to evolve, to grow, and to change. We are now immersed in the information age where knowledge awaits our every curiosity, where information lies patiently, waiting to be discovered, and true wisdom is but a mouse click away. This fascination with life, health, and the human sprit has inspired me to write this book. As a Fitness and Lifestyle Management Consultant, I have become quite fascinated with teaching people, not only how to change their bodies, but also how to change their hearts as people all over the world are now beginning to see what we, in the fitness community, have seen all along.

As we all begin to approach health and fitness with more of a balanced perspective, only then can we begin to achieve our true physical potential. This approach to wellness begins to free people from their need to achieve a certain weight, or even look a certain way. The fact is that this gift of life that we have all been given needs to be cherished, not simply quantified by scales, calories, fat grams, or dress sizes. In our ever–so–diligent quest of perfecting an ideal body image that is neither healthy nor real, millions of people have succumb to the temptation of diet pills, quick fixes, and overnight exercise programs.

What this book and my career are all about are building stronger lives, one body at a time. In fact, I have dedicated my career and my life to teaching people how to live healthier, stronger, and happier lives by providing easy–to–understand information about health, fitness, nutrition, and lifestyle change. The fact is that this book comes at a time when billions of dollars are being spent every year on "miracle" products, diets, and ideas that are potentially dangerous and extremely misleading to say the least. The unfortunate truth is that there are currently no organizations that regulate the weight–loss industry or the misleading claims that several of these companies are making. For that reason, there comes the need for some regulation, a watchdog of sorts, to "keep an eye" on what these companies are promising, and what they are most likely not telling us. This is a job that I have decided to embrace and I thank all of you for allowing me the opportunity to do so.

Believe me when I tell you that my own frustration with the weight–loss industry comes from asking thousands of questions of these self–proclaimed "experts" and not receiving the answers that I was so desperately in search of.

Clearly, there will never be a consensus regarding anything related to fitness, nutrition, or weight loss. There are hundreds of different diets and exercise programs gracing the pages of magazines and books, headlining news stories and talk shows, and being promoted in health clubs across the country. Not surprisingly, each one of these methods all seems to contradict one another! What this does is it leaves millions of people chasing their tails as they try desperately to find the answers to their health and weight–loss questions.

With the barrage of information currently available to us, the responsibility that we all have as health and fitness consumers is to arm ourselves with as much information as possible. This knowledge comes, not only about exercise and dieting, but also about ourselves. This self–awareness will enable all of us to begin establishing a foundation as to who we already are; not simply whom we think we may someday become following the next quick fix. Bear in mind that as valuable and effective as self–exploration may be, the acquisition of knowledge does not imply a thorough understanding by any means. How many people do you know realize exactly what they need to do to change their lives, but for whatever reason, fail to do anything about it? Research has proven the life–long benefits of a healthy diet and exercise. Research has also proven that smoking destroys our lungs, high–fat diets destroy our hearts, and extreme alcohol consumption destroys our liver. Apparently, knowledge is not always power, is it?

The fact is that being thin has become all the rage in today's extremely idealistic and self–absorbed culture. This obsession with constant dieting and compulsive exercising has proven to be the foundation of a yet another cultural epidemic. With the incidence of eating disorders increasing each year, it has become apparent that we all need to begin approaching our health from more of a balanced perspective. Time To Stop Dieting and Start Living will provide you with that perspective! In fact, in reading this book, you will become aware very quickly that, despite the inclusion of various tips and strategies related to health, fitness, and weight loss, this is not simply a "how–to exercise" or a "how–to lose weight" type of book. What this book is about is helping you become aware of who you already are without all of the dieting and exercising. This book is also about changing, not who you are, but changing the way you see yourself. Therefore, by the end of this book, you will learn to approach your health and fitness from a more fundamental perspective and as such, it will enable you to approach your life in a completely new way.

This book is just the beginning of a life–long

journey and I congratulate each one of you for taking the first step. Enduring success in anything begins with a decision to take control and the desire to take action. For making that decision to once and for all, take control of your lives, you should be commended greatly. The time to invest in your future is now and I would like to ensure you that your investment has been wise. In fact, I have no doubt in my mind that you can change your life if you simply decide to do it. I am truly committed to helping you learn what it takes to permanently transform your lives, and I will do whatever it takes to share my knowledge with you.

The pages that follow represent years of individual study and research that has proved invaluable in my own life and can do the same for you. Throughout this book, I will share with you the information that was provided to me along my journey. I hope that this information is only the beginning of a lifelong journey of health and fitness in your own lives. Good luck!

PART I

GETTING STARTED ON
CHANGING YOUR LIFE

"Nothing splendid has ever been achieved except by those who dared believe that something inside of them was superior to circumstance."

—Bruce Barton

1
Taking Charge of Your Health

Before we begin our journey together, it is important that we discuss what change is and where it comes from. I think it's safe to say that each one of us wants to change something in our lives, right? Whether it's our body, our hair, our career, or our relationships. It just seems like most people, for whatever reason, feel like whatever they have in their lives right now is probably not good enough. Although this constant search for self–improvement is an admirable quality, when it comes to trying to change things about ourselves, this self–defeating mindset tends to elicit self–perpetuating feelings of inadequacy.

With the emerging popularity of self–improvement seminars, books, and audiotapes comes the realization that our problems are not unique. People from all over the world are experiencing exactly what we are, maybe in a slightly different context, but we are all the same! The quest for the perfect body has, and will continue to inspire people to climb higher, jump farther, and run faster than ever before. In fact, for hundreds of years, people have been searching for the most effective ways to transform their bodies. The question is, how far are you willing to go to get there?

Before you can begin to take control of your health, your first objective is to come to the realization that YOU are responsible for getting to where you are right now! That means that you are also responsible for getting to where you want to be! Bear in mind that things don't just happen to us without some underlying cause. We are not all just governed by chance, simply waiting for things to happen as they will. We do have control here, and now is the time that we all start taking responsibility for our own health. My question to you is this; how badly do you want to change, and what will it cost you if you don't?

The fact is that far too many people make excuses about why they don't have to change something about their life, when they know they desperately need to. Remember that before change can actually happen, we first need to take responsibility and acknowledge the fact that we did in fact cause the problem and that we can change if we want it bad enough. True wellness is determined by the decisions that we make about how to live our lives, not only by our circumstances or the "cards that we have been dealt."

In spite of the countless number of reasons

people come up with for why they are unable to change something about their health or their body, not surprisingly, there are very easy things that we can all do that can make measurable improvements in our overall health and well–being. If you have family history of heart disease or stroke, eat well, exercise, and learn to manage stress. If you have family history of obesity, monitor caloric intake and exercise regularly. If you have family history of alcoholism, drink in moderation. If you live in a highly polluted area, don't smoke. The list goes on and on! The point is that we have a lot more control over our own health than some people would like to think.

Interestingly, despite their need to achieve their own idea of physical perfection, not surprisingly, most people are not willing to do the work necessary to achieve their health and fitness goals. The desire for instant gratification keeps people from taking the small steps necessary to achieve enduring success. So what happens? Well for one, people go on diets, they start taking miracle fat burner pills, and they buy into some "5–minute a day" exercise program and wonder why their lives never change!

Realize that the first step in changing anything in your life is first, deciding exactly what it is you want to change, and then doing something about it. You would be surprised at just how many well–meaning people proceed to talk about the new diet or exercise program that may one day change their lives. The problem is that, as they say, talk is cheap! In actuality, when it comes to your health, not taking action will actually cost you a lot more than just taking action in the first place! Have you ever heard how much it costs to recover from a heart attack?

Aside from health and fitness, when it comes to our "real lives," some people can't decide on anything because they are fearful of making the wrong decision. They don't put the pressure on themselves to make decisions quickly, and inevitably, out of fear of failing, they just keep things the way they are. This fear of the unknown keeps people from making the changes that may very well save their lives at some point in the future. Therefore, as you begin to explore your health and the various ways you can improve it, bear in mind that you have to be willing to work hard to achieve the success that you are after. With that commitment to yourself and your health, you are beginning to pave the way for a lifetime of physical vitality and enjoyment.

2
Define Your Purpose

It has been said that the starting point of all achievement is first and foremost, defining your purpose. Setting goals for yourself sets in motion a series of events that is neither fully understood nor completely appreciated. Being able to harness this power of decision enables people to project themselves into the future and visualize their lives how they would like them to be.

Of course, goal setting requires a certain level of commitment and time and your part. As with any new skill, goal setting needs to be something that you practice daily! One way to start developing your "goal setting muscles" is to start making "to–do" lists every night before bed. Getting into the habit of writing something down that you need to accomplish the following day and actually getting it done, creates a sense of excitement that will, more often than not, improve your long–term goal setting techniques.

The simple act of writing your goals down on paper turns a seemingly passive wish into a burning desire that will drive you to produce results that you never dreamed possible. Writing your goals down creates a sense of accountability far beyond simply stating your goals out–loud. In doing this, you are activating more senses and as such, making these goals more real and that much more compelling. Of course, changing your eating and exercise habits is a bit more significant than "doing laundry" or "washing dishes." However, once you establish the habits when the responsibilities are less significant, making the larger, more important decisions in your life will be that much easier for you.

The fact is that beginning any exercise and nutrition program is going to take a lot of work and a significant amount of planning. In terms of your health, defining your purpose is not only important, but without a clear vision of what you are striving for, how will you ever know if you are on track? Too many people live day by day, expecting things to just fall into their laps, without taking the initiative to do whatever it takes to succeed. They approach their lives with a sense of expectancy and utter complacency that is hardly conducive to producing the results they are after.

Realize that getting into the habit of goal–setting can and will pay tremendous dividends in every area of your life if you are willing to try it. When you are ready to start setting goals for yourself, here are a few strategies that will help you along the way:

1. Plan ahead: By developing a very clear understanding as to where you currently are as well as where you would like to be, you are providing yourself with the direction you need that will help you produce explosive changes in every area of your life! In being honest with what you already have, what you want, and what you are willing to do to get there, you are beginning to set the stage for long–term success.

2. Create a recipe for success: For the same reason that you wouldn't attempt to cook something new without following a systematic set of instructions, you shouldn't expect goal setting to be any different. As with anything else, success is quite predictable and it can be duplicated if you follow the steps necessary to succeed.

3. Be realistic: In beginning to set goals for yourself, an important point is that while setting your sights high is an excellent idea, not surprisingly,

there are those who have extremely unrealistic expectations of themselves. What this does is guarantee frustration! Instead of walking up to the plate and trying for the short grounders, these people expect a homerun every time they are at bat. Why? The answer to that is simple; people want results, and they want them fast! Unfortunately, what most people spend a lifetime destroying, they expect to fix overnight.

4. Start small: By taking on smaller goals first, (only eating fast food twice a day instead of three times a day for the next week), and then tackling the bigger goals next (going to the gym two to three times a week), you are minimizing the likelihood of becoming overwhelmed or discouraged. The only way to reinforce your new behavior is to make sure that you allow yourself the enjoyment of achieving these smaller goals first before you move on to the bigger ones. To do this effectively, reward yourself with a new outfit, a new pair of shoes, or some other tangible object that you can see

every day. What this does is remind you of the fact that you did in fact reach your goals successfully. While there are things like massages or fancy dinners that can be just as much of a reward, although effective, after these rewards are over, there is no physical reminder of what you have accomplished.

5. Turn up the heat: Just as professional basketball players can miraculously sink the winning shot at the buzzer to win the championship game, you too can create the same sense of urgency for yourself. Give yourself a deadline and stick to it! Something amazing happens when you introduce a self–imposed deadline in that this level of tension will often elicit a competitive fire in you that you may have never been aware of.

6. Believe in yourself: You have to know, with every ounce of conviction, that you have everything inside of you right now that you need to reach your goals. You might not realize how you are going to get there,

but as long as you know that you will not accept failure, you can and will find a way! Simply light the competitive fire inside of you and refuse to accept defeat!

7. Be persistent: In attempting to achieve any health goal, please don't expect to see results overnight, because you aren't going to. In addition, don't give up if things don't go exactly as planned because they aren't supposed to. Just remember that achieving anything worthwhile is not going to be easy. You are going to have to work, and work hard to get there. The question you need to ask yourself is, "How badly do I want this?" Because if your goal is powerful enough, you will do whatever you need to do to succeed.

As you can see, anything you want is within the realm of possibility, as long as you are willing to work hard to achieve the success you are after. As with anything else, there is a definite art to setting goals. Goal setting is not merely something that is reserved for a select group of people. There are successful people who will say that their success is a direct result of their hard work and dedication. Some will even admit that they were in the right place at the right time. However, the one thing that all successful people have in common is that at some point, whether it was instrumental in helping them become successful, or a key factor in helping them stay successful, every single one of them will tell you that without their vision, they would have nothing. So just look towards the future, keep working hard every single day, and I promise you that success will be right around the corner!

3
Ask and You Shall Receive

"He who asks the questions cannot avoid the answers," "Once the student is ready, the teacher will appear," "Seek and you shall find;" as common as these simple phrases are in our language, it still seems apparent that people either don't believe them, or they just don't listen!

That said, my question is this: Why would anyone walk into a gym or start a nutrition program and expect to know exactly what they're doing? That's like saying, "You know, I need to have this tumor removed from my brain, but I think I can do it myself." Every single day I hear people brag about just how much they know about nutrition and fitness, yet none of them seem to be doing anything about it!

Remember that there are people who spend years learning particular skills so we all don't have to. They call this specialization of labor! In fact, there are those of us who spend years in college and countless hours in the "real world" learning the art of health, fitness, nutrition, and lifestyle change. What this means is that there are definitely people who you should consider consulting with before jumping into anything. That means that if you have questions about your diet, go see a registered dietician. If you have a question about starting an exercise program, go see your doctor. If you want to learn proper exercise techniques, hire a personal trainer. The point is that there are very qualified people out there who can help you achieve whatever it is that you want in your life, you just have to take the initiative to ask them. Don't try to do everything by yourself! There are professionals out there who have already done the work for you! Believe me when I tell you that they will be very happy to help you, so don't be shy! Just take a deep breath, swallow your pride, ask the right people the right questions and you will be surprised at just how much time and effort you can save!

4
Expect Ups and Downs

Have there ever been days in your life when you have felt unstoppable? Days where you have been "in the zone?" Times when everything you touched turned to gold? Absolutely! Have there also been days when you couldn't even make a sandwich without lighting your house on fire? Of course! The point is that when it comes to your health, there will be days when you will be making amazing progress. You will be stronger than ever before, you will be able to eat whatever you want and not gain weight, and everything you do will seem to work out perfectly. It should not be surprising to know that there will also be days when you will barely be able to drag yourself through the day, let alone your workout!

Assume that, on a Monday, you had a great morning, an energetic day, a powerful lunch packed with just the right nutrients, and you just found out that you won the lottery. Most likely, you are going to have a great workout that day. That Wednesday, let's assume that you decide to do the same workout you did two days earlier. Let's just say that you had a horrible morning, a sluggish day, your spouse just left you, you had to eat fast food for lunch, your dog just died, and your car broke down. Do you really think that you are going to be stronger than you were during your last workout? In fact, when you try to lift more weight than you did during your previous workout, not only will you be increasing the likelihood of injury, but you will also become extremely frustrated and discouraged. The point is that you are only as strong as your body is in that moment. Inevitably, this will vary each time you exercise, so be prepared for the ups and downs.

In order to create lasting changes in your life, specifically with your health, you have to expect obstacles along the way. A common mistake is to begin an exercise or nutrition program and expect everything to run smoothly. Big mistake! Obstacles are going to show up! Therefore, it's better to expect these ups and downs, and welcome the message that they may be bringing with them.

5
Learn to Manage Stress

Do you realize that more than half of everyone you will ever meet in your lifetime will, or have experienced some health–related problem associated with increasing levels of stress? The fact that approximately half of the people in this country are "stressed out" in their homes, their jobs, and in their relationships has proved that stress is rapidly becoming yet another cultural epidemic that is very real, and extremely deadly!

Since stress has become so common in today's high–intensity and fast–paced culture, there comes the need to develop a certain level of understanding as to what stress is, what causes it, and how to deal with it when it inevitably shows up in your life. Knowing that there are different types of stress, each with different causes, can prove invaluable in learning effective coping techniques that may some day save your life.

The word stress actually means "any physiological response to anything that disturbs our bodies normal functioning." Events such as taking a test, experiencing a death in the family, cutting your finger, exercising, even being kissed for the first time; all of these events inevitably cause some physiological change in our bodies and are therefore considered as "stressors." Interestingly though, stress is traditionally thought of as something that seems to "happen to us," as if it were some disease that just happens to fall into our laps without warning. As you will see, our response to stress is quite predictable and in most cases, can actually be controlled.

As most people have heard of before, there is something called the "fight or flight response" we all experience when dealing with some stressful situation. Personally, when I first heard the term "fight or flight," I didn't think it was the most appropriate way of describing a situation where I was neither planning on fighting anyone or flying anywhere! The point is that this response is in fact, very real and the physiological changes that happen within our bodies are also extremely powerful!

Not surprisingly, the same hormonal and physiological changes that result from the fight or flight response also tend to precede the majority of heart attacks. During a stressful situation, our heart rate and blood pressure increase to supply our muscles with the oxygen and nutrients they need to help us "escape" that particular situation. Blood clotting is also increased as the body is preparing itself to repair any cuts that may occur during the "encounter." Among the other physiological changes that occur during the fight or flight response, these changes specifically, over the long term, have been known to contribute to the development of cardiovascular disease. Since this ultimately causes significant damage and weakening of the heart, as you can imagine, dealing with stress will significantly decrease your chances of developing heart disease.

Another set of health concerns that are widely accepted as "stress–induced" conditions are the different digestive problems associated with high stress levels. When we experience stress, stomach acid production increases dramatically. Aside from the immediate reactions to this (stomach pain, digestive problems, and heartburn), in the long term, this elevated acid production may eventually lead to the development of an ulcer. Interestingly, several over–the–counter antacids are being sold to help relive the symptoms of heartburn (band–aid approach), instead of addressing the underlying stressors that caused the problem in the first place!

Headaches are another common condition in those people who are experiencing abnormally high levels of stress in their lives. During stressful situations, blood is being re–routed to the working muscles by squeezing down on the blood vessels that are leading to the "non–important" areas of the body. As with the stomach, during the fight or flight response, blood is being re–routed from the brain which may ultimately cause the majority of tension headaches associated with stress. Not surprisingly, over-the-counter as well as doctor-prescribed "headache remedies" are essentially covering up the real issues by counteracting the squeezing effect of the blood vessels in the brain. Much like an antacid, this band–aid approach is only covering up the real problem, and as such, this method is hardly conducive to restoring the body's normal physiological functioning.

Those experiencing high levels of stress also have a difficult time sleeping. Have you ever noticed how difficult it is to fall asleep the night before a big exam, or minutes after an argument ended with your significant other? Why is that? Remember that the stress response is preparing us for battle. The last thing that your body will allow itself to do is to sleep whenever you feel threatened.

In addition, several other conditions such as anxiety, panic attacks, nervousness, muscle tension and aches, tremors, fidgeting, irritability, impatience, hostility and anger, difficulty concentrating, fatigue, and depression have all been reported in those who experience high levels of stress in their lives. Is that to say that stress causes all of these conditions? Maybe, maybe not. The point is that experiencing stress in your life is definitely not going to help prevent these conditions from developing either!

Not surprisingly, in recent years, the amount of doctor–prescribed medications has virtually eliminated the need for effective coping strategies. Whenever someone feels a bit uneasy in their lives, the first thing they are expected to do is run to the doctor for the next quick fix. From pain medications used to alleviate headaches and stomach problems, antacids to relieve heartburn, sleeping pills and anti–depressants to help people momentarily forget all of their problems, to anti–anxiety drugs to help people relax; what each of these well–meaning doctors are forgetting is that pharmacological interventions are only covering up the real issues! In fact, these band–aid approaches to health care may actually be making people's problems worse!

Again, in working with people to help them achieve their health goals, all of these issues need to be addressed. Before I can start helping people change their lives, we first need to address the underlying cause of whatever it is they are trying to change. Once we determine the underlying stressors in people's lives, we can then begin approaching health and fitness with a clearer perspective, which, in turn, translates into longer lasting success.

6
Enjoy The Journey,
Not Just The Destination

After years of working with people with every possible health concern you can imagine, one thing has become very clear to me. In my experience, I have found that there are only two types of people in this world; there are "destination people" and there are "journey people." Without exception, everyone I have met in the fitness arena is either one or the other, with very few individuals who have some combination of the two.

When it comes to their health, "destination people" are very goal oriented and they are extremely committed to achieving their fitness goals. Not surprisingly, these individuals will do whatever it takes to succeed, at any cost. These people have no problem exercising seven days a week, they count calories, they don't eat after a certain time, they don't eat before a certain time, they go on bizarre diets, and they generally live their life in a "fitness bubble". Unfortunately, destination people seem to be more likely to develop eating disorders and other health problems associated with chronic dieting and exercising. They become locked into a lifelong obsession with a certain fitness goal, be it weight loss, or whatever it is for them. As would be expected, these individuals are everywhere!

On the other hand, "journey people" are more free–spirited when it comes to their health. These are more carefree individuals who could care less about where they end up, they just love the journey. These people don't count calories, they don't care how much body fat they have on their bodies, they eat whatever they want (within reason of course), and they are generally more easy-going when it comes to their health. These people have fewer eating disorders, they are typically easier to be around socially because they don't mind "cheating" occasionally, their biggest monthly expense isn't from the health food store, and they are usually "regular" people who happen to stay healthy.

Not surprisingly, in our extremely idealistic and weight–obsessed culture, there are far more "destination people" than there are "journey people." In the past several decades, people have become so obsessed with calories, dress sizes, fat grams, and everything in between, that they are actually becoming more unhealthy every single day. Despite the origin of this cultural epidemic, it is critical that people begin enjoying the process of being healthy, not just the potential of becoming healthy at some point in the future.

Again, my job is not promoting a certain physical ideal that is neither healthy nor realistic. My goal is to teach people how to incorporate fitness into their lives, not make fitness the foundation of it. The last thing that I want to see is people spending three hours a day in the gym while going on some bizarre diet because they feel they "have to." For this reason, in working with "destination people," we first need to determine their underlying "issues" with weight and their own self–image. At that point, we can then begin to set an appropriate course of action that best fits their lifestyle.

That leaves the important question; if I am a "destination person," how do I become a "journey person?" Well, that question should arouse some serious thought about your own self–image and why you feel you need to do what you do. Whether you deprive yourself of your favorite foods, or go to the gym every day of the week for hours at a time, you have very specific reasons that make you feel obligated to do these things. Your job is to figure out why you do them.

Remember that obsessions about fitness and dieting are only visible signs of deeper issues that need to be addressed. As with any eating disorder, with chronic dieting and exercising, there is usually a perceived lack of control. This causes people to feel that they need to re–gain that control by whatever means possible. For some, that means going on diets, for others, that means spending hours in the gym every day. It just seems like too many people are expecting diets and exercise to fill some gap in their lives that isn't being filled by other means.

Bear in mind that our lives are only as strong as the foundations that make them up. Without that foundation of self–esteem, confidence, and inner strength, everything that you will ever work for will be taken from you. From your body, to your career, to your relationships, without a strong sense of who you already are, at some point or another, you will lose everything! Once we address the underlying body–image issues and resolve them, we can then begin to incorporate good nutrition and an active lifestyle into people's lives.

PART II

WEIGHT LOSS AND WEIGHT CONTROL

"Imagination is more important than knowledge."

-Albert Einstein

7

The Secret to Lasting Weight Loss!

Now that I have your attention, to the dismay of millions of people around the world, the secret is that there truly is no secret! There is no one right or wrong way to approach weight loss. What most people do is spend a lot of time, money, and effort trying figure out the secret to losing weight as quickly, and with as little effort as possible. Instead, they should be spending more time trying to figure out why they gained the weight in the first place!

In order to effectively and consistently lose weight, we first need to understand the physiology of weight gain. Since one pound of body fat contains 3,500 calories, in order to lose one pound of fat, you need to avoid these additional 3,500 calories, either by burning them off with exercise, or by not eating them. It's that simple! Now, if your weight loss goals are higher than one pound a week, just do the math. For example, if you want to lose two pounds of fat this week, then that's 7,000 calories that you need to either burn off or not eat during the next seven days.

Now to put that into perspective, in order to

lose two pounds in the next week; try eliminating 1,000 calories every day for each of the next seven days. That's a lot of calories! Trust me when I tell you that by the end of the week, you will not be a happy camper. Now try losing ten pounds of fat in one week! That's 35,000 calories in seven days! Most people can't do that in a month, let alone one week! The point is that whenever you hear of some miracle diet that guarantees that you will lose any more than two pounds in one week, think about how much of that weight really is fat, and how much is actually water weight and lean muscle.

The question that you may still have is; Don't I need to count calories if I want to lose weight? Some say yes, others say no. For most people, it would seem like quite the chore to live their lives with a calculator and a measuring cup in their pocket! It is true that, in order to lose weight, we need to be consuming fewer calories than we are normally accustomed to eating. However, this does not imply that we need to start counting every calorie we eat! Therefore, without providing you with a series of numbers as to the "right" amount of calories each of us needs to consume every day, the bottom line is this:

- If you are gaining weight, you are eating too much

- If you are losing weight, you aren't eating enough
- If you are maintaining weight, you are eating just the right amount

Real scientific huh? Do you see how easy this can be? So without giving you meaningless numbers as to the exact amount of calories you need to be eating every day in order to lose weight, just realize that if you aren't losing weight, you are simply taking in more calories than you need, period! Weight loss does not have to be as complicated as counting every calorie you eat and writing everything down either. So despite what most people think, eating carbohydrates, eating late at night, or eating fat in their diet does not necessarily make them overweight! Essentially, over–eating anything is the main reason people gain weight. Therefore, instead of counting every calorie, just judge by results, how your clothes feel, how you feel, and the rest becomes easy!

8
The Truth Behind Weight Gain

In order to maximize the weight loss experience, we need to spend some time trying to determine why people overeat in the first place. For the most part, I think we can all agree that there are five styles of eating, each serving its own purpose and each playing its own distinct role in the manifestation of weight gain.

The first type of eater is referred to as a functional eater. Functional eaters approach their meals with a definitive purpose, and that purpose is to fuel their bodies. Their meals are typically more nutritionally balanced, they take less time to finish, and they involve fewer calories with a lower incidence of overeating. Functional eaters typically spend a considerable amount of time planning their meals, they go shopping on very specific days of the week, they carry lists with them when they go food shopping, and they usually designate an entire day for cooking as they prepare meals for the entire week. As would be expected, these individuals are typically leaner and healthier. However, while this is an admirable way of approaching their nutrition, some of these individuals tend to become obsessed with the process of "eating healthy." These people won't eat before or after certain times of the day, they won't eat certain things because it's "against the rules," they don't eat out as often as they would like to, and they tend to drink more meals by virtue of meal replacement shakes.

On the other side of the feeding spectrum, there are social eaters. Social eaters tend to eat at parties, they eat out four to five times a week, and they tend to eat just for the sake of eating. These individuals might not even be hungry at all, but they tend to eat just because "it's the polite thing to do." Social eaters tend to be more easy going about their health and usually don't care about what's "right or wrong" when it comes to their diet. As would be expected, social eaters are prone to becoming overweight and they usually have the hardest time in shopping situations as well.

The third type of eating style is boredom eating. Boredom eating, as the name implies, is eating when you have nothing better to do. The best thing to do to avoid this type of feeding trigger is to just do something! If you have to leave the house to prevent yourself from eating, go ahead and leave the house! If you need to go to mall and just walk around, then go for it. The point is that once you realize that being bored is a feeding trigger for you just find something to do that keeps your mind off eating!

The fourth type of eater is a convenience eater. Convenience eaters will eat as long as there is a relatively small investment of time and effort in doing so. These people usually avoid cooking at home and tend to eat fast food or frozen, pre–packaged meals from the supermarket because of the ease of preparation.

The last eating style is emotional eating. The emotional eater tends to eat when they feel depressed in some area of their lives. They may have lost of a loved one, they may have just broken off a long–term relationship, or they may have just lost their job. Whatever the cause, just remember that eating at peak emotional times is not only a bad idea, but it is arguably the most instrumental cause of weight gain.

Bear in mind that I am not saying that any one of the five eating styles is any more beneficial or harmful than the others. In figuring out what type of eater you are, you will gain valuable insight as to what may be causing you to overeat. Remember that the real key to any successful weight–control program is identifying and modifying the very behaviors that are contributing to the weight problem to begin with.

9
Stop Dieting and Start Living!

Interestingly, the word "diet" has become so passé in our self–absorbed vocabulary that it has become somewhat trendy. From movie stars to models to "regular" people, "chronic dieters" seem to constitute a good proportion of the American population. My question is this: Why do so many people go on diets? What is it about a diet that people love so much? Is it the pleasure of depriving yourself of exactly what you love the most? How about forcing yourself to eat foods that you wouldn't eat even if you were paid to do so? Is it the tasty powder mix that you have to drink three times every day? Or how about eating the delicious meal replacement bars that you'd much rather use to plug the leak in your bathtub?

What if I told you that all diets are completely ineffective and potentially dangerous, would you believe me? What if I told you that each time you go on a "diet," you were actually making yourself fatter? Well, believe it! Instead of making minor adjustments in their lives, "chronic dieters" tend to periodically go for the "homerun" by trying the next new diet craze. In this case, not only will dieting not be effective for them, but I would almost bet that no matter how hard they try, and how much weight they do lose with each successive attempt, they will have to continue dieting for the rest of their lives just to maintain their current weight. What are we missing here?

In working with people, most of them are surprised to hear that, in our initial meeting, that if they want to lose weight, they need to eat more. What they are assuming is that they now need to consume the same amount of calories during each meal, and now eat more of these meals. While this might be a great idea if becoming a sumo wrestler was in your future, it is hardly conducive to losing weight!

When I tell people that they need to eat more if they want to lose weight, what I am actually saying is not that they need to eat more calories throughout the day. What I am saying is that they just need to eat the same (maybe fewer) calories, and simply eat more frequently throughout the day. The problem with eating five to six times every day is that people are not distinguishing between a "meal" and an "eating session." Meals are usually much larger, they contain more calories, and they are typically referred to as breakfast, lunch, and dinner. Compare that to an "eating session" which is usually a fraction of the calories of an entire meal. This technique is one of the most overlooked in the area of weight loss because it is assumed that, in order to lose weight, fewer calories need to be consumed. While this is true to an extent, answer this question; if you were eating 2,000 calories every day, which do you think would be easier for your body to handle, two "meals" of 1,000 calories each, or five "eating sessions" of 400 calories each?

To illustrate just how ineffective dieting really is; have you ever noticed how a grizzly bear can eat once, hibernate, and still manage to sustain life for months at a time? Do you realize how they do this? Their bodies know that after they eat once, the nutrients that they just ate need to keep them alive for a significant amount of time afterwards. Since body fat is an extremely efficient source of fuel, the food eaten by the grizzly bear is converted into fat quite rapidly. The body fat that is now being created and stored enables all of the normal metabolic processes to continue without requiring additional nutrients. In this case, eating so sporadically will cause a significant decrease in overall metabolic rate, not only because of the lack of nutrients, but also due to the lack of energy resulting from the caloric deficiency. Does this very thing happen in the human body? Absolutely!

For those people skipping meals in an attempt to lose "weight," the fact is that eating fewer times throughout the day is only teaching your body to become fatter! Avoiding meals throughout the day is just the beginning of the adaptive process that will invariably occur within the human body. Without eating every few hours, the body has no idea when the next meal is coming. In an attempt to protect itself against starvation, as soon as you do eat, your body will begin to convert the food into unhealthy body fat! Remember that our bodies don't care where or how they get the energy they need to function. Our bodies are built to carry on very specific tasks with or without the help of the food we eat. Better we learn to help our bodies do its job because if you don't help, eventually, the body will break down!

The unfortunate truth is that people are expecting diets to help them solve all of their problems. Let's face it, diets are not the end all to our happiness, they won't eradicate our troubles, nor will they eliminate the cause of our unhappiness. Not surprisingly, in order for a change this significant to last, we first need to address the underlying issues that cause the overnight binges and "cheat days" before we look for the next way to cover up the problem. And in case you haven't realized it yet, diets are only temporary solutions to long–term problems! What we need to understand is what causes people to become overweight, not just the way to make them thin again.

Therefore, instead of going on a "diet," just start incorporating regular exercise and healthy nutrition into your everyday lifestyle instead of periodically "going for the homerun." Not only will this help you stay on track, but you will also be less likely to feel cheated and deprived. Remember that our bodies are very revealing about what they want, and they will do whatever they can to "tip us off" to whatever they need. If you find yourself struggling to find the energy to exercise, before reaching for the "energy pills," take an honest look at what you've been eating throughout the day. You would be surprised at how easy it is to pinpoint what your body may be missing if you have the courage to look for it. Just don't ignore these cravings because if your body needs something, you will suddenly feel a craving for something that you should consider addressing.

10
Weight Loss vs. Fat Loss

How many times have you ever heard someone bragging about how much weight they've recently lost? Maybe they started exercising, maybe they went on some bizarre diet. However they got there, they are just thrilled that they lost all of that weight! As a fitness consultant, I hear this every day! Inevitably, whenever I do hear someone inform me of the dramatic amount of weight that they recently lost, the first thing that I usually ask them is where they think the weight came from. After they look at me with a blank stare, as I seem so unimpressed with such a miraculous achievement, I go on to explain to them that weight loss does not always equal fat loss! In fact, up to this point in the book, I have been referring to fat loss and weight loss interchangeably. By the end of this chapter, you will see that they are indeed, very different.

In an ideal world, every ounce of weight that we shed from our bodies would be fat weight, not simply water weight and lean muscle. In the real world however, this is hardly the case. The key to remember is that body weight can be lost from muscle, water, and potentially fat. Therefore, saying that twenty pounds of weight loss all came from fat is extremely idealistic and unfortunately, not always the case. The rule of thumb is; the quicker the weight was lost, the less likely it was to be fat. And despite what most people think, "weight" really is easy to lose. We all have muscle weight, organ weight, bone weight, a few extra limbs, and a lot of water weight floating around in our bodies that will be more than happy to go. Just remember that it is the fat that causes the health risks, the heart attacks, the high blood pressure, the "pooch," and the beer belly, not the weight, per se!

The bottom line is that we need to reevaluate what "weight loss" means, our reasons behind it, and the lengths we are willing to go to see the scale weight go down, while causing our health risks to increase exponentially. In fact, the multitude of health benefits of losing excess body fat can all be eradicated by implementing a risky, unhealthy, and potentially dangerous weight–loss plan. So just throw the scale away, start making small changes in your diet and exercise program, and your fat–loss effort will become a permanent change to a new life!

11
Exercise Is Not The Only Answer

Not surprisingly, when people reach a point in their lives where they will no longer accept their current health status, one of the first things they want to do is start exercising. Certainly, as a fitness consultant, I do promote the value of participating in regular exercise in order to achieve and maintain good health. However, the majority of people are assuming that exercise is the only answer, which, as you will soon see, is only one small piece of the puzzle.

When I began working as a personal trainer, the majority of the work that I did with my clients was done in the gym. People would come to me with a list a mile long about what they wanted to change about their bodies. At that point, my job would be to teach them proper exercise technique and develop a set of workouts for them that I was sure would help them achieve their health goals. Unfortunately, after months of working with several of my clients, despite how hard they were working in the gym, I started noticing that their bodies weren't changing. At that point, I realized that there was something I was missing and I was determined to discover what it was.

For years, I was investing everything I had into teaching my clients everything I knew about health and fitness. After several years as a personal trainer, unfortunately, I was becoming quite disenchanted, as were my clients, with the lack of progress that some of them were making. What I eventually realized was that I was placing too much emphasis on our "gym time," and not enough emphasis on our "real life time." Because of this, quite early in my personal training career, I was forced to accept the fact that my clients' success or failure had little or nothing to do with me, but more to do with their own effort when they left the gym. As difficult as that was for me to accept, at that point, I began to appreciate the importance of healthy living, not only healthy exercising.

For those people who spend a good amount of time in the gym, bear in mind that just because you do exercise, that doesn't mean that you should be eating fast food and drinking beer every night because you feel that you've earned it! Not surprisingly, there are people who go to the gym three or four days every week just so they can "make room" for the junk food that they plan on eating! Remember that exercise is merely one small piece of the puzzle and it should not be expected to be the end-all to your health. There are other decisions in your life that need to made consistently that will have as much, if not more of an impact on your life than just the time you spend in the gym. Once you begin using exercise as a tool to achieve better health, and not the only means by which to achieve it, then and only then will you be able to take your life to the next level.

12
Stop Blaming Carbohydrates!

In the spirit of the emerging "anti–carbohydrate" revolution of the past decade, it is only fitting that we address some of the more popular diets and weight–loss programs that are out there and why they should be avoided. Without mentioning the names of the specific diets, I think it's extremely important that people realize that the creators of these anti–carbohydrate diets are physicians, not dieticians! Now, don't get me wrong, I think doctors are fantastic healers, but they do not study nutrition in college! That seems odd to me considering the fact that people are taking nutrition advice from people who have virtually no training in nutrition!

Without getting into specifics, let's just touch on what happens when people go on a low–carbohydrate diet. Premature fatigue becomes a common complaint in those consuming too little energy–rich carbohydrates. More often than not, those people on low–carbohydrate diets need to take energy pills and drink coffee just to get them through the day. Why is that? Well, for one, protein is not intended to provide energy, carbohydrates and fats are. Therefore, when your body has to provide energy without the right fuel necessary to do so, I promise you that it will get it from somewhere! In fact, by consuming too little carbohydrates, your overall metabolic rate decreases which will ultimately increase your body fat storage!

Since fat and protein both slow digestion down, when people are eating high protein/high fat diets, since they feel "full" for the majority of the day, they are unable to eat the five or six smaller "eating sessions" necessary to maintain an active metabolic rate. As a consequence, contrary to popular opinion, eating a diet too high in protein and too low in carbohydrates may actually cause muscle to be lost and fat to be gained! When carbohydrates and fat are not providing energy, muscle tissue will inevitably be sacrificed to provide the body with what it needs to sustain normal functioning.

In addition, whenever anything is removed from your diet, specifically carbohydrates, you are going to become deficient in some very important nutrients. Interestingly, the various anti–carbohydrate diets insist that the reduction of foods like pasta, rice, grain products, fruits and vegetables, natural juices, and bread will guarantee a dramatic decrease in body weight in an extremely short period of time. While this is true to an extent, remember that since carbohydrates promote water retention, when they are removed from the diet, water weight will be lost fairly quickly. What a diet like this does is cause the scale weight to decrease, thus reinforcing the extremely misguided notion that carbohydrates are "bad." What this means is that if you find yourself losing any more than two or three pounds every week, believe me when I tell you that you are losing water weight and lean muscle, you are not losing fat! The implications of this are that I have seen 120–pound women who, by body–fat standards are considered clinically obese! How? Again, losing weight and losing fat are completely different. And losing "weight" does not guarantee that you are becoming healthier either!

There are also potential long–term health risks associated with consuming a diet too high in protein and too low in carbohydrates. The increased acid production caused by excessive protein consumption has been thought to contribute to gastric and esophageal ulcers. The lack of fiber associated with a diet low in carbohydrates may contribute to the development of colon cancer and ultimately, heart disease. Kidney and gallstones may also develop due to the buildup of toxins associated with high protein consumption.

As you can see, there are very specific reasons why a low-carbohydrate diet should be avoided. Again, the take–home message from this chapter is balance. My mission here is not to bash all of the diets that have seductively found their way into millions of homes across the country. What I am concerned with is making sure that you understand that just because a particular diet is effective, it does not mean that it is good for you. Remember that in almost any "diet" situation, most of the weight lost during these and the majority of the other extremely short–term "deprivation situations," is water and muscle weight, not fat weight! The bottom line is that any diet that tells you that you can't eat foods that are completely natural and better yet, indispensable to human life, you should consider avoiding!

13
Forget The Food Guide Pyramid

Have you ever glanced on the back of a food label and noticed a big triangle with a bunch of pictures of food lying inside of it? This is what has been coined the "Food Guide Pyramid." This wonderfully impractical invention provides a simple "guide" as to the appropriate amount of nutrients we need to be consuming every day. Here's the problem that I have with the Food Guide Pyramid: The fact that people from all walks of life, carrying very different body weights, incredibly different amounts of body fat, all with very different dietary needs and dietary restrictions, all of whom have very different activity levels, are all being advised by the Food Guide Pyramid to eat 2,000 calories a day! What exactly does that tell us?

Is that to say that every human being walking the face of the planet has exactly the same dietary needs? Does the Food Guide Pyramid assume that all of us need exactly the same amount of carbohydrates, the same amount of vitamin D, and the same amount of fruits and vegetables every day? Unfortunately, this is exactly what the Food Guide Pyramid does! The fact is that each of us has very different dietary needs that are not being addressed within the geometric confines of the Food Guide Pyramid. For those people who have very specific dietary needs, I strongly recommend that you seek the advice of a registered dietician if you have questions that you need answers to. Because as the name implies, the Food Guide Pyramid is simply a guide that can and should be modified to fit your own unique lifestyle.

14

Eat Right Before You Go Shopping

Have you ever noticed that you always end up buying more food than you need to whenever you shop hungry? Better yet, doesn't it also seem like that the junk food aisle seems a lot more appealing whenever you've gone too long without eating? Why is that? Well, there are very specific things that trigger the sensations of hunger, and those things are very different for different people. The most powerful trigger to begin eating is, of course, the sensations of hunger.

Typically, when we haven't eaten for several hours, our blood sugar levels begin dropping quite rapidly. This is one of the reasons why we suddenly develop a craving for "sweets" whenever we haven't eaten for some time. What this instinctive response is doing is looking for the quickest and easiest way to restore your normal blood sugar levels. Since the brain functions primarily on carbohydrates, whenever you do crave something relatively sweet, bear in mind that your body is trying to tell you something!

Therefore, in order to avoid those inevitable visits to the junk food aisle, do yourself a favor and not only eat something right before you go shopping, but try eating something relatively sweet. What this will do is cause a fairly sharp spike in your blood sugar levels, which ideally will prevent a sudden lapse in judgment that we all are guilty of making at the supermarket!

15
Make Healthier Choices

Butter or margarine? Ice cream or frozen yogurt? Low fat or fat–free? One percent or skim? The truth is that there are so many food choices that people are being forced to make every day and for the most part, people have no idea what the best choices really are. In fact, a good number of people make the mistake of trying to give up the foods they love because they feel that it's the right thing to do. Not surprisingly, the fastest way to fail at a weight–loss effort is giving up the foods you enjoy. That will only make you feel deprived and more likely to relapse. Just make healthier choices!

What this means is that if you love ice cream, buy the frozen yogurt instead. If you love hamburgers, make them yourself instead of going to the fast–food restaurant. If you love fried foods, bake instead. And for those people who refuse to give up certain foods, that's fine too. In fact, you don't even have to give up your "cheat foods," simply eat them less often.

One simple technique that I have taught to help people make healthier nutrition choices is what I call the avoidance technique. What the avoidance technique assumes is that if you have certain weaknesses, maybe for chocolate, maybe cigarettes, whatever it is for you, just don't buy it! Despite the simplicity of this idea, you would be surprised at just how effective it can be if you use it consistently. Imagine when you wake up in the middle of the night and reach for your favorite junk food and it's not there. Guess what? No guilt! Then again, if you really want the chocolate–covered doughnuts in the middle of the night, I suppose you could get dressed, get in the car, drive all the way to the 24–hour supermarket, stand in line, get back in the car, drive all the way back home, and eat them then. Most of the time, the inconvenience of having to do all of that will prevent most people from "cheating!"

The point is that you have complete control over the health decisions that you make every day! Remember that choice, not circumstance, will ultimately determine the quality of your life and whether or not you are an example of good health, or yet another alarming statistic of just how destructive our poor decisions can be!

PART III

BECOMING AN EDUCATED
HEALTH AND FITNESS CONSUMER

"No greater lesson was ever learned than by the
man who truly searched for the answers."

-Adam Bordes

16
Take It From Who It's Coming From

Can you count how many different weight–loss commercials or advertisements you have seen in your lifetime? Do you recall just how many of them insist that they have invented the very thing that has eluded you and the rest of the world for years? Every single day, within the pages of health and fitness magazines and late–night infomercials, some new company is boasting about their brand new discovery that is neither new nor is it worth bragging about!

With the ever–increasing availability of nutrition and fitness information, it is becoming even more important than ever that we begin assessing the validity and credibility of the various sources of this information. Because let's face it, making sound choices about your health is becoming increasingly more difficult. As we all have been exposed to at some point, there are several different sources of health, fitness, and nutrition information available to us. From books, television, magazines, to the health food store, every day, we are all being bombarded with information that is neither a healthy nor a safe means to achieve any of our health goals.

Interestingly, all of the self–proclaimed "experts" in the fitness industry have a unique challenging to overcome. First, in order to elicit more business, it is essential that they disprove and discredit everyone around them to make themselves appear more knowledgeable. They use their bodies to imply an understanding of health and fitness that may or may not even be there. Finally, after convincing their prospective customers that everyone else has no idea what they're talking about, they need to begin promoting their own potentially inaccurate information. The truth is that there are so many different opinions out there, and not surprisingly, all of them seem to contradict each other!

From a marketing perspective, bear in mind that the weight–loss industry is, and will continue to be one of the most lucrative businesses in the world. In order to sustain this business, companies spend billions of advertising dollars every year trying to create a feeling of need for various products and ideas where no real need exists. How do they do this? For one, they pay superstar athletes and entertainers millions of dollars to use (or at least say they use) certain products. What do you think that does for the demand for their products?

In fact, several years ago, a man we all

knew and loved was paid a substantial amount of money to become the spokesman for a certain product. The company used this man's superstar status to create a demand for a product that he wouldn't even hold in his own hand, let alone use! The company knew that if the buying public, as naïve as we all were at the time, saw this man appear in commercials for a product that he wouldn't even use, they could make billions of dollars. Any guesses? The product was Pepsi and the man was Michael Jackson! Speaking of Michael's, do we really think that Michael Jordan eats Ballpark hot dogs? He might. What I do know is what happened to annual sales once he started telling the world he did!

Manufacturers of fitness equipment and the creators of "miracle" diets realize that to sell their products, they need to reassure us, the buying public, that we can in fact achieve the results that we want, without having to work for them. While this is an excellent way to sell products, this is not the most effective way to create healthier lifestyles.

The fact is that companies are designing products that require little or no effort on our part mainly because they know these products will sell. Being that the our culture is frowned upon and thought of as one of the most inactive cultures in the world anyway, these fitness companies are creating products that are conveniently filling that particular need promoting more results for less work. We live in a society of fast food, remote controls, take–out, microwaves, instant pudding, and several other things that were truly designed to make our lives easier. Despite the convenience provided by some of these "modern technologies," the unfortunate truth is that we have things we do and use every day of our lives that have made many people complacent and inactive. The implications of this are that people are becoming more unhealthy than ever before, and we are all inevitably bearing the personal and economic burden of preventable disease and disability.

Interestingly, despite the multitude of different promotional techniques and sales gimmicks, the majority of the companies within the fitness industry all seem to have one thing in common. Television commercials, magazine articles, and various other advertising mediums all seem to promise us the same big results with a considerably smaller investment of time and effort. From nutritional supplements to home exercise equipment, it seems as if the majority of these companies are making promises that they simply cannot stand behind. In fact, the majority of these companies are spending billions of advertising dollars each year trying to convince us that the bodies that we've spent our entire lives destroying can be transformed in minutes a day. This is exactly why people are frustrated! People are expecting to see overnight results that are just not possible!

Despite the complete saturation of "overnight" miracle products and diets, there are still very dedicated people who make exercise and a healthy diet a significant part of their everyday lifestyle. Unfortunately, despite all of their hard work and dedication, some of these individuals, for whatever reason, are still not where they want to be. The remainder of the buying public is being convinced that they can avoid exercising and eating healthy, exercise for five minutes a day, eat whatever they want, take a miracle "fat burner" pill, and miraculously have a healthy, strong, and fit body. What these companies aren't telling us is that everything comes with a price; our careers, our homes, our relationships, and yes, our health is no different.

The bottom line is that we need to find an easier way to change our lives without involving diet pills, ineffective home exercise equipment, or risky diet plans. Although it is possible to receive helpful health information from television, books, or magazines, remember that just because a particular diet or exercise program helped someone on TV or in a magazine lose fifty pounds, it does not guarantee that it is a safe or effective way for you to achieve the success that you are after.

17

Determine What Works For You

One day, you walk into your local bookstore and eagerly approach the health and fitness section. Upon your arrival, you begin your search for the book that will provide the answers to all of your health and fitness concerns. After several hours of relentless contemplation, you find exactly what you've been looking for. This is it! You've found the book that will help you go from where you are today to exactly where you want to be! After opening the book and briefly glancing over the chapter titles, you soon begin to feel an overwhelming sense of excitement. You've hit the jackpot!

The more you read, the more you wonder how your life has come this far without this priceless information! In fact, as soon as you arrive home, you plan on using every bit of this information, word for word, until you achieve all of your health and fitness goals. At that point, you realize that you are on your way to living happily ever after!

As bizarre as this scenario sounds, does this happen in real life? Absolutely! People with very good intentions walk into bookstores and open up books or magazines that provide very general information to millions of eager people. Is all of the information misleading? Absolutely not! What is misleading is assuming that everyone reading the information is actually capable of using all of it.

Remember that these magazines and books are providing very general, "cookie cutter" information that may be appropriate for some, but is definitely not appropriate for everyone. Saying that everyone should be avoiding carbohydrates, or exercising a certain way, or that everyone should be doing, using, or eating anything, is only half of the truth. Bear in mind that any commercial weight loss or fitness program is simply a guideline that should be investigated for safety and effectiveness and should not always be followed as if it were the only way. The point is that we all need to find whatever it is that works for us.

18
The Truth About The Body Fat Test

Recently, I was working with one of my regular clients at a national health club chain in Atlanta. Having noticed that most of the other trainers were conducting body fat tests fairly regularly, I became somewhat intrigued as to what the buzz was about. Having extensive laboratory practice with two very specific methods of measuring body fat, I was interested in how this "new" method worked. The interesting thing was that, of the countless number of different methods of measuring body fat, I had not only never seen this one before, but I had never even heard of it!

Following a brief instructional, I decided to attempt the "new" technique with one of my own clients. After we finished the test, I was quite surprised to find out that her percentage of body fat was significantly higher than what I had originally anticipated. After trying to console her for almost an hour, I reassured her that body fat tests are only as accurate as the technique and the person conducting the test. Not surprisingly, that was the last time I heard from this woman! What does this tell you? Apparently, this woman placed a significant amount of importance on the results of a test that means relatively little in the overall scheme of things. She allowed something that should not be an issue, to become an issue, and as a result, she forgot why she started exercising in the first place.

Over time, I started noticing that, after having their body fat tested with this new method, more and more people were approaching me with somewhat of a depressed look on their face. Each time I asked them what was wrong, they all told me that they were upset at he amount of body fat they had on their bodies. When I asked them what their body fat percentages were, every one of them told me numbers that were quite staggering to say the least. When I asked them how it was measured, they all admitted that they were tested by the same "new" method. After watching an excessive amount of people suffer through the humiliation, I decided to take the test myself. To my surprise, according to the results of this particular test, my body fat measured almost twice what I was accustomed to. It was then when I started asking questions, because now it became personal! After asking club management why they thought the numbers were reading so high, I was not prepared for what I was told.

Not surprisingly, when someone becomes extraordinarily upset with their current health status, they are going to do whatever they can to relieve the situation. One of the managers of the club informed me that, when people hear just how much fat they have on their bodies, they are going to be more likely to join the gym and ultimately, hire a personal trainer. This technique (not the testers themselves) seemed to be giving people an increased body fat reading in an attempt to elicit more personal training revenue! Needless to say, I was furious! In an attempt to generate more business, the company that designed this machine did so in order to deceive people into thinking that they were "fatter" than they actually were! What this does is it creates a sense of urgency as people are now doing virtually anything to achieve their health and fitness goals, namely hire a personal trainer at the gym. From a marketing perspective, this is an excellent idea! However, from a personal perspective, this scam clearly demonstrates just how little truth is being provided to the millions of health and fitness consumers across the country.

Remember that quantifying our lives by virtue of body fat percentages, dress sizes, fat grams, and calories immediately puts you in "destination mode" and will ultimately cause more harm than good. Reducing the amount of body fat on your body is an excellent starting point as you begin an exercise and nutrition program. However, when you start "chasing numbers," be it a specific body fat percentage, or a specific weight you would like to achieve, you are essentially missing the point of becoming healthier in the first place!

19
Buying a Membership To a Health Club

During the past few decades, home fitness equipment and exercise videos have virtually exploded onto the health and fitness scene. Why the increasing popularity? Part of the answer comes from the fact that these products are being sold to people who either have no time or desire to make the dreaded hike to what is now becoming more of a social freak show than an opportunity to get in shape. In fact, exercising at home has become quite the norm for many people.

Despite the popularity of these "home—exercise videos," the fact is that the last thing that most people want to do at home is exercise. If people actually do exercise at home, I would say with complete certainty that the majority of them will exercise at home for a few weeks and eventually get bored or simply give up. Therefore, the only other option is to become a member at a health club. Not surprisingly, choosing a health club can be a royal pain in the neck! Unless you know what to look for, you could lose a lot more than your money.

Most people, being the eternal skeptics that

we are, encounter an eager salesperson at a local health club and naturally resist their efforts to sell us a membership. Why is that? Well, while they are in business to make money, why is it that people will resist the very thing that may potentially save their lives at some point in the future? The bottom line is that whenever people do get past the initial resistance of "locking themselves into another long–term commitment," there are a few things you can do to ensure that your "health club experience" will be as enjoyable as possible. Therefore, for those people who are ready to join the ranks of the "fitness elite," there are a few things to keep in mind before making your decision.

Before you decide to begin a tour of virtually every gym in town, save yourself the time and effort by asking your friends and coworkers where they have memberships. In addition to the location of the health club, ask them what they like and dislike about the club they belong to. Believe me, they will be more than happy to tell you! Once you get a few ideas about the different gyms in town, make sure that you have some idea of what you're looking for in a health club before you get there. If you want to be able to work with brand new free weights, keep that in mind. If you're looking for an extensive line of exercise machines or cardiovascular equipment, remember that too. The point is that if you come across a club that looks appealing, but doesn't have anything that you plan on using, there's no sense in getting a membership there, is there?

Once you've developed a few good leads, you need to go visit each club. When you walk in, tell them that you're visiting and you'd like to be taken on a tour of the club. Let them take you on their tour, that's their job. Once the guided tour is done, let them know that you'd like to take a second look around on your own. Remember that you're in charge here, not them, and you need to walk in with the confidence that demonstrates that. Once they leave you to yourself, you need to walk around and inspect every part of the health club, especially the parts of the club they may not have shown you on their tour. Occasionally, salespeople will conveniently avoid some of the weaker parts of the club. While this is an extremely effective way to sell memberships, it is also important that you see every part of the club that you are about to invest in.

Another thing you may want to consider doing is examining the equipment very carefully. While there are some clubs that clean every piece of equipment every night, as would be expected, there are some that don't. Therefore, before you sign a contract, during your own tour of the facility, notice any rust, discoloration, missing pieces, or missing handgrips on the equipment. Bear in mind that if the gym won't take care of a $5,000 piece of equipment, how concerned do you think they're going to be with you and your $40/month membership? Think about it...

After your tour of the facility, you may want to consider walking up and introducing yourself to someone. Even though you may not know anyone when you get there, simply walk up to one of the members, introduce yourself, and let them know that you are considering becoming a member. Ask them what they like and dislike about the club. In fact, the people who are getting involved with every aspect of the facility are the ones who can tell you about the aerobics schedules, the credibility of the trainers, the cleanliness of the facility, and the overall "rating" of the club. What better way to "avoid reinventing the wheel!"

Once you feel satisfied that you have seen the entire club, the equipment doesn't look like it can be sold for parts at the junkyard, you've spoken to a few people, and you feel confident that this is the right club for you, go home! That's right, walk out! Remember that just like buying a car, purchasing a long–term membership at a health club is highly variable and more often than not, very negotiable. As would be expected, at the end of your tour, it is likely that one of the salesmen is going to tackle you, grab on to your leg, and not let you leave without a fight! That's fine! After they ask you into the sales office (which they will), just let them know that you would like to continue looking around to see the other clubs before you make your decision. Most salespeople will respect that and in fact, once they know that you are still not "sold" on their club, they may even throw in a few "extras" in a last–minute attempt to try and "sweeten the deal." Therefore, even if you fell in love with the club, you are absolutely sure that you want to purchase a membership there, and despite the fact that you may not even want to see any other club, remember that the key here is to not look too eager!

Purchasing a long–term membership at a health club is going to be a decision that you are going to have to live with for a long time. Invest the time now and your experience at the health club you have chosen will pay enormous dividends, both physically and emotionally, for years to come.

20
Hiring a Personal Trainer

As with choosing a health club, hiring a personal trainer can be even more of a challenge! While there are trainers out there who are committed to helping you succeed, there are others who are very content spending more time talking than actually helping you. For those who are helping you, there are very specific things you can do to help ensure that your fitness experience is beneficial to you, and not only to their bank account!

Before we talk about what it's like to work with a personal trainer, just remember that no one in his or her right mind wants to hire one! Having a trainer in and of itself does not guarantee that you will achieve the body of your dreams either! People make the mistake of assuming that, once they start working with a personal trainer, their bodies are going to change miraculously, without doing any work. That's not going to happen! In fact, what I tell people is that the typical personal trainer works with their clients three out of the 168 hours every week. My clients realize that the bulk of our work together happens whenever we leave the gym, not as soon as they walk in.

When people are paying for a certain amount of a personal trainer's time, they are not only paying for a cheerleader, someone to count repetitions for them, or someone to talk to! What they are paying for is the hope that they will receive the information that will help them achieve their ideal body at some point in the future. The responsibility of a personal trainer is to recognize that and do their best to develop a comprehensive roadmap that helps their clients get from where they are now, to where they want to be in the safest, most cost-effective, and fastest way possible. The personal trainer's job is to teach their clients how to get the most effective workouts by doing something they enjoy and something they will continue doing for a lifetime.

Once you are ready to begin working with a personal trainer, before you choose randomly from a pool of trainers you may have never met before, call your health club and ask to speak with the personal training coordinator or the fitness director. These are the people who decide which trainer would be best for a particular client based on the client's time or gender preferences, if the client has a medical condition that most trainers can't even pronounce, etc. Once a trainer has been chosen for you, now is the time to ask for credentials! Unfortunately, there are individuals who are employed by health clubs across the country who aren't even certified to be training people, let alone legally allowed to be paid for it! There are also people out there who happen to have excellent physiques who carefully avoid the education and certification issue by promoting their bodies and their "experience." Remember that, just like any other profession, there are very specific guidelines for becoming a personal trainer. Unfortunately, these guidelines are not being met by everyone.

After finding out that the trainer is certified, remember that there are fitness organizations that are more credible than others. Saying that a trainer is "certified" doesn't say much. However, knowing who certified them is a completely different ball game. That being the case, you need to find out who certified the particular trainer so you can investigate the credibility of the organization before you begin working with them. (There are certified personal trainers who have proved to be nothing more than good test takers who want a weekend job. The bottom line is that a certification is by no means a guarantee of skill or ability as a personal trainer).

Once you find out who certified your personal trainer, call the organization or visit their website in order to find out exactly what is expected of its certified members. This is important because different fitness organizations have very different certification requirements and it is important to know that if you are diabetic, have recently had reconstructive knee surgery, are taking medication for high blood pressure, and are nursing a herniated disk, you aren't seeking the advice of someone who lacks in the appropriate training or experience.

In addition to finding out what kind of experience the trainer has, it is also important to know what they studied in college. Along with, and even more important than the certification issue, you deserve to know what their educational background is before starting. Being "certified" is one thing, but having a degree in some health–related field says a lot more. And for those people who say that "real world" experience is more important than education in becoming a personal trainer, I would bet that they're trying to justify their lack of education! Assuming that is true, if "experience" is just as good as a quality education, let me ask you this: If you went in to have brain surgery, who would you rather have behind the knife, someone who went to school for ten years, or someone who took a study at home course for six weeks? Think about it!

Another equally important question that you need to ask yourself is what the personal trainer charges for their time. It is important to remember that, as you've seen, choosing a personal trainer involves several things that go beyond the price of their services. However, when it does come down to price, you really do get what you pay for. While there are some trainers out there who have no problem charging you $100/hour, there are also those who only feel comfortable charging you $20. So if you're only willing to pay $20/hour, don't be surprised when you ask your trainer to tell you the benefits of exercise with diabetes, and he or she responds, "dia—what?"

Assuming that you went through all of the steps outlined here, and you feel comfortable with the trainer that was chosen for you, go ahead and book the appointment. However, if you don't feel comfortable with the particular trainer, be it the lack of experience, education, or whatever else, let the personal training coordinator know. At that point, they should do whatever you need them to do in order to best meet your individual needs. If they can't accommodate you, take your business elsewhere.

While I do understand that this whole process may be a bit challenging for some people, think of it this way: You wouldn't hire someone to work for your company without seeking references, knowing their educational background, and understanding their objectives for employment. Why should your health be any different? The truth is that there are virtually thousands of different approaches that a personal trainer can take to help you achieve your fitness goals. Hopefully, they are doing their best to design customized fitness programs that are specific to your needs, not only their own!

21
Does Your Trainer Make The Grade?

After some serious thought and consideration, you've finally chosen a personal trainer. After you meet for the first time, there are several things to keep in mind as you begin your journey together.

- When you first met, did they do more talking than listening?

  The fact is that your first meeting together is your time! This is when you need to be addressing your concerns, your goals, and exactly what you hope to get out of your time together. Be aware of premature promises and notice if they spend more time talking about what they can do for you, as opposed to listening to what you want to accomplish.

- Are they truly interested in where you would like to be with your health? Or are they more interested in training you how they want to train you?

  While there are personal trainers who seem genuinely interested in helping you, there will be others who are more interested in increasing their clientele with a complete disregard for your health. Remember that if your trainer doesn't ask you what your health goals are, how else will they know how to customize a fitness program for you? If that is the case, be sure to let them know up front what you're looking to do and how you won't accept anything else.

- Are they actually explaining why you're doing something? Or do they have the "Just do what I say" attitude?

Is your personal trainer taking the time to explain the importance of performing weight-bearing exercise in the prevention of osteoporosis? Are they teaching you how cardiovascular activity helps prevent high blood pressure?. Are you learning the different resistance training techniques and why some of them are safer than others? Remember that you hired a personal trainer so you can learn about fitness, you didn't hire someone to count repetitions for you.

- Are they taking the time to teach you about fitness? Or are they deliberately keeping valuable information from you so you have to keep paying them for their time?

  Most personal trainers will provide you with helpful information for the sheer benefit of helping you change your life. However, if you notice that your trainer is simply "teasing" you and leaving out important information be-cause they want you to keep coming back to them, be sure to leave out the "renewal clause" in your next months contract!

- Are they trying to prove how smart they are?

  While I do explain to my clients that strengthening the back and abdominal muscles is important in maintaining good posture, I do not talk about the unique length–tension relationship between the agonist–antagonistic pairs within the thoracic cavity! The chal-lenge of being a fitness professional is finding the best way to translate seemingly worthless information about anatomy and exercise physiology, physics, biomechanics, and sports nutrition, applying it, and explaining how it all applies to our clients' lives. Using big words about the body might be impressive to someone who cares. For someone who just wants to fit into their clothes, they could care less!

As you can see, hiring a personal trainer can be a bit more painless if you follow the steps outlined here. Once you discover exactly what it is you are looking to achieve with your health, finding a qualified fitness professional can be one of the most important decisions you can make so choose wisely! Remember that you are hiring the personal trainer, not the other way around. Since they are working for you, you need to assess their credibility before you begin paying them for a service that they may not even be qualified to provide.

22
The Truth About Supplements

Meal replacements, protein powders, fat–burners, energy pills, metabolic enhancers; These are just a few of the more readily available "dietary supplements" on the market today. With the growing emphasis on dietary supplementation, the questions that you should be asking yourself are: What is a dietary supplement anyway? Who should be taking them? Who shouldn't be taking them? Are they safe? Will taking them really improve my health? Can taking them actually impair my health?

In recent years, the term "sports nutrition" has become somewhat of a buzzword in the fitness industry. Health and fitness magazines are promoting products that are designed for active individuals who may be deficient in some very specific nutrients. What these companies are implying is that, for whatever reason, active people may not be providing their bodies with the nutrients they need to function efficiently. The implications of this are that people are being convinced that they need to begin taking nutritional supplements to "pick up" where their inferior diets left off. The question that people need to begin asking themselves is, "Do I really know enough about these particular supplements that I am putting into my body?" When I ask people that question, they respond like a robot, repeating exactly what they were told at the health food store or in the magazine. More often than not, people have no clue what they're putting into their bodies.

Essentially, there is no way of knowing how a particular dietary supplement will react with your body. We are all made differently and what may work very well for one person may cause some catastrophic event for someone else. The point is that, as the warning labels indicate, "Dietary supplements are not evaluated by the Food and Drug Administration, and they are not intended to diagnose, treat, or cure any disease." What that means is that you need to supplement at your own risk! Dietary supplement companies are promoting potentially inaccurate information mainly because they can make millions of dollars doing so! Just remember that if a dietary supplement is extremely expensive, especially when compared to the cost of "ordinary foods," you need to ask yourself how "necessary" the supplement really is.

23
The Truth About Protein

In recent years, protein–based supplements have become the dietary supplement of choice among bodybuilders and fitness enthusiasts alike. Everyone seems to speak with confidence about how protein builds muscle, but it seems interesting that there are several other functions that protein serves that all seem to take a backseat to the "protein builds muscle" theory. In fact, despite being an extremely important component of our physiological health and overall well–being, the "back–seat" functions of proteins such as enzyme, hormone, and antibody production, fluid and electrolyte balance, as well as acid–base balance, are all being conveniently overlooked. Despite the fact that these functions are not only extremely important, but they are also critical to sustaining life, few supplement companies are going to announce: "Improve your acid–base balance and ensure adequate hemoglobin production just by taking Protein Power 2000!" Remember that the buying public is going to be told exactly what it needs to hear, which, in this case, is only half of the truth.

What also seems interesting is that within various fitness and bodybuilding magazines, you will have no problem finding several articles discussing the roles of protein in the manifestation of muscle growth. Is that to say that protein isn't important in building muscle? Absolutely not! Because when we exercise, yes, we do need more protein! But, we also need more carbohydrates and fat! Remember that when we become more physically active, we need more calories across the board, not just from protein! Foods rich in carbohydrates and fats are extremely cheap for us to buy at the supermarket. This is exactly why supplement companies are promoting so much protein, because they make more money that way!

The bottom line is that, despite what all of the bodybuilding magazines are promoting, all of the protein we need, whether we are weekend warriors or elite athletes, resides very nicely in a nutritious, well–balanced diet. In fact, the majority of the time, a balanced diet really can give our bodies exactly what they need. If and when there are any nutrient deficiencies present, a good multivitamin can't do us any harm. But when your frequent shopper miles from the local vitamin supply store offers to fly you to Hong Kong and back forty seven times, I would seriously reconsider your dietary options! The moral of the story is that there is much more to protein than just muscle growth. So just eat a balanced diet, save your money, and take it easy on the supplements!

PART IV

BEGINNING YOUR EXERCISE
PROGRAM

"The human body is the best picture
of the human soul."

-Ludwig Wittgenstein

24
Exercising For Maximizing Fat Loss

In designing exercise programs for people of all ages and fitness levels, specifically cardiovascular exercise, every single person that I have had the opportunity to work with has one thing in common. Each one of them wants to know how hard and how long they need to exercise in order to maximize fat loss. In fact, the majority of commercial cardiovascular fitness equipment presents a chart that indicates that there are two very distinct training intensities. The first intensity is referred to as the "cardio zone," and the other is referred to as the "fat burning" zone. What this is implying is that exercising at a very specific level will be more effective at increasing your cardiovascular health, while the other is more beneficial at burning fat.

In fitness, a common misconception is that in order to "lose fat", you must exercise at a lower intensity for a longer period of time. This lower training intensity is commonly referred to as the "fat burning zone" and represents approximately 55-60% of maximal effort. My question is this; are they implying that any intensity above or below this so–called training "zone" is completely ineffective at burning fat?

What is true is that during lower intensity exercise, a higher percentage of calories that are burned are coming from fat. However, when you exercise at higher intensities, although the percentage of calories coming from fat decreases, overall caloric expenditure increases which translates to a greater amount of fat loss. What this means in English is that during low intensity, aerobic exercise, the majority of calories (50%) are coming from fat. Let's assume that during your walking session, you burned a total of 200 calories. What this means is that, of the 200 calories that was burned during the exercise session, 100 of those calories (50%) came from fat sources.

Now, assume that you were running for the same amount of time. Let's assume that instead of 50% of your calories being burned from fat sources, let's assume that because of the higher intensity of running, you are now only burning 35% of your calories from fat sources. At first glance, this may not seem like the ideal situation if maximizing fat loss was your goal. However, when you look closer at the total amount of calories being burned, this paints a much clearer picture as to which is more beneficial to you.

Assume again that instead of walking for 20

minutes, you decided to run for 20 minutes. In this particular case, you are now burning 400 calories instead of the previous 100. Although now, while only 35% of your total calories are coming from fat, in the end, you are actually burning 140 calories from fat, which is 40% greater than before!

As you can easily see, total energy expenditure is the most important factor for maximizing fat loss. What that means is that in order to lose fat, you must simply use more calories than you are taking in and you will lose all the fat you want. In terms of choosing an exercise intensity that works best for maximizing fat loss, the choice is yours because in the end, you will burn the same amount of calories. Low intensity exercise does have its merits, but it should not be chosen as the basis of a so–called "fat–burning" principle.

25
Muscle Does Not Weigh More Than Fat

Here's a question for you; which weighs more, a pound of gold or a pound of feathers? They weigh exactly the same, right? That said, the old adage that "muscle weighs more than fat" is not true! A pound is a pound is a pound! What is accurate is saying that muscle is more dense than fat because it is a bit more compact, and thus appears to "weigh more." Bear in mind that when you start exercising, you are potentially going to gain weight. Don't panic! Although the scale reveals that you are gaining weight, just know that, while the scale weight may be increasing, remember that you are increasing lean muscle and decreasing body fat simultaneously, which is exactly why you started exercising in the first place!

Not only does muscle not weigh more than fat, but muscle does not "turn into" fat either! Have you ever avoided exercising because of your fear that if you ever stopped, your muscle would turn into fat? What about the time that you did stop exercising and you happened to gain weight around your midsection? Has this ever happened to you? If it has, you're not alone. But if it makes you feel any better, muscle cannot "turn into" fat, they are two completely different things! That's like saying that if you leave water around long enough without using it, it would turn into oil! That will never happen! The fact is that when we are actively involved in a fitness and nutrition program, the lean muscle on our bodies will (ideally) burn the fat that surrounds it. When we stop exercising, it's the inactivity that's actually causing the fat gain, not so much the lack of resistance training per se.

26
Don't Be a Hero In The Gym!

Contrary to popular belief that "to increase muscle size, you need to lift heavy weight," it's important to remember that muscles will grow in response to their perception of effort, not yours! What that means is that, instead of lifting heavy weights to prove yourself, why not use less weight, but actually control the weight and not throw it around? Now I realize that everyone believes that "to get big muscles, they need to lift heavy weight." However, when using proper exercise technique, you would be surprised at how much less weight people can actually lift! In addition, by using less weight with more control, not only will you be minimizing the likelihood of injury to your body, but you'll also be minimizing injury to your ego when you need to take six weeks off from a severe muscle tear! Simply create a fitness program that enables you to train with the most intensity with the least amount weight, and you will be amazed at how much more your body will respond!

Here are several different ways that you can increase the intensity of your workouts without increasing the amount of weight you are lifting:
- The first way to increase the intensity

of your workouts is to just slow down! Correct me if I'm wrong but it seems like the majority of people lifting weights seem to have ants in their pants! Why are they going so fast? You would be surprised at how much more difficult each repetition becomes when you increase the amount of time during each repetition.

- The second way to increase intensity is to increase the number of sets or repetitions during your workouts. By increasing either the number of sets or repetitions, or both, you are instantly increasing the intensity of your resistance–training workouts and thus decreasing the need to increase the amount of weight you are lifting.

- The third way to increase the intensity of your workouts is by decreasing the amount of rest time between sets. Remember that rest time should be used for recovery, not social hour! While I do realize that workout time can be quite interactive, just keep in mind why you are in the gym in the first place. While you shouldn't be anti–social, you are there to work!

That means that if you find yourself resting more than two minutes in between sets, you are probably wasting time and need to arrange to meet whomever it is you're talking to later at the bar!

- The fourth way to increase intensity is to add additional exercises to your workout. While there are people who seem inclined to do four or five different exercises for each body part, you really only need to do one or two. If you notice that, after trying the first three techniques for increasing intensity, that your workouts are still fairly easy for you, just add one more exercise for every body part, not five!

- The fifth way to increase intensity is to maintain perfect form. Although some people are impressed with those who throw hundreds of pounds around in the gym, I'm sure not impressed! As I tell people, if they can still lift as much weight as they've been lifting without "cheating," then I would say that they need to increase the weight. However, for those people who are cheating, it's time you leave your ego at the door, lighten the weight, and do the exercises the right way!

Remember that the reason we do resistance-training exercise in the first place is to become stronger and prevent injuries in our "real life," while not causing more harm than good in the gym. If you find yourself working through pain and straining muscles during your workouts, try using the techniques outlined here. With these techniques, not only will your workouts be a lot more fun, but you'll also be minimizing the likelihood of injury.

27
Take a Vacation From Exercise

How many people do you know exercise every day of the week? What about 5–6 days every week? For those who do, remember that whether you're doing cardiovascular training, resistance training, or both, the body perceives them both as physiological stressors! Not surprisingly, whenever your body doesn't feel like doing whatever it is that you are about to subject it to, it will shut down! This usually translates into sudden injury, sickness, or overall fatigue.

In order to see results from your resistance-training workouts, you need to give your body enough rest time to allow adequate healing between these workouts. Now I know this will be tough for some people, but the only way to actually see results is to give yourself enough time to recover. Therefore, if you don't want to get sick or randomly pull a muscle, just give your body the rest it needs and I promise you that you'll see better results that way. In fact, have you ever been exercising and just ignored that stabbing pain in your back? What about the time you were doing squats and your knees starting sounding like a Rice Krispies commercial? While I do understand the whole obsession with killing your body in the gym, if something starts hurting, or if you start feeling nauseous, lightheaded, or dizzy during your workout, just go home! Interestingly, people constantly brag about this as if they should be congratulated about how intense their workouts are! Remember, feeling pain or sickness during your workouts is not a good thing. When that does happen, your body is trying desperately to tell you something so why not listen and go home!

Something that I usually do myself and recommend to my clients is taking one whole week away from exercising every four to five weeks. For those people who occasionally reach a strength plateau with their workouts or fail to see improvements with their body, a week away from the gym may be answer. What this does is it causes a certain "de–training" effect that will intentionally cause the muscles to "forget" what they are normally accustomed to doing.

To illustrate this idea, let's assume that, when you start exercising, you can lift fifty pounds. After approximately six weeks of resistance-training, let's assume that you are now capable of lifting one hundred pounds. More often than not, the dramatic increase in strength will eventually plateau and in fact, you may even become "stuck" at one hundred pounds for weeks at a time. In this case, I would take approximately one week away from the gym. Upon your return, you notice that, instead of being able to lift the one hundred pounds that you lifted during the last workout, you are only able to lift seventy pounds. While this is a significant strength decrease, once you look closer, you are still forty percent stronger than you were when you started exercising in the first place! Interestingly, after you begin your resistance–training program again, you notice that you quickly return to your "pre–vacation" strength and in fact, surpass the previous plateau of one hundred pounds.

Remember that you have to give your body the time that it needs to recover and become stronger. Your body doesn't care about the wedding dress or the bathing suit you want to get into next month, nor will it have any compassion for you when you start over–training either. Much like a well–anticipated and well–deserved vacation from work, you will be amazed at how much more intense your workouts will become if you occasionally reward your body with a weeklong vacation!

PART V

THE FUTURE OF YOUR HEALTH

"Some men see things as they are, and say
'Why?'
I dream of things that never were, and say,
'Why not?'"

-George Bernard Shaw

28
Have Fun!

How many people can actually say that they enjoy exercising? What about walking on a treadmill and feeling like a rodent on a hamster wheel? I bet that excites you! Despite a certain level of enjoyment that a lot of people do feel while exercising, it just seems like too many of them walk into their workouts three or four times a week and dread every second of it. What a waste! In their defense, I do realize that not everyone enjoys being in the gym. It does take a very special type of person to stare at themselves in tall mirrors while wearing clothes fitting for a strip show!

What I am suggesting is that if you like walking, walk; if you like playing softball, play softball, if you despise going to the gym, you don't have to go to the gym! The point is that once you find something you do enjoy, do it, do it often, and be consistent! Remember that the right health and fitness program will be its own incentive, while poor choices will turn exercise into a chore that will be avoided. Therefore, the most effective way to ensure that you continue with your new lifestyle is by doing something you enjoy.

29
Failure Is Not An Option!

The fact is that more than eighty percent of the people who attempt to accomplish anything are going to fail the first time! What does that say about them? Does that mean that they are failures? Does that imply that there is no hope for them? Of course not! Just think of anything you have in your life right now: the home you sleep in every night, the relationships you now have with the people around you, the successful business you now operate, or the car you drive every day; did they all come easily? Did they all come the first time you worked for them? Absolutely not!

Think of it this way; we wouldn't plan a vacation for months, pack the car, drive for a few days, run into a detour, and say, "Forget it, let's go home!" That would be ridiculous! Unfortunately, this happens every single day! There are people who make plans to achieve some health and fitness goal, begin working towards that goal, run into an obstacle, get frustrated, and simply give up. This is crazy! We need to expect obstacles, welcome the lessons they bring with them, and we need to know what to do with them once they do show up.

In terms of your health, no matter how many times you have attempted to lose fat, change your diet, quit smoking, or whatever else, and "failed," don't lose hope! The reason most people fall short of reaching their goals is not because of a lack of will power or desire, they simply do not have an effective strategy to help them succeed. In fact, most people think of previous attempts to change their weight, their eating habits, or their exercise routines as failures. When in reality, each "miss" potentially provides valuable information about what made a difference and what didn't. Your job is to figure out what worked well, what didn't, what was going on in your life when you became bored or frustrated, change whatever you need to change, and keep trying until you succeed!

Once you do figure out what you want in your life, that is when the real work begins. Saying that you want something to happen in your life is a great start, but again, talk is cheap! While trying to sound as optimistic as possible, I think we can all agree that whenever you attempt to do anything new in your life, the possibility of not succeeding is there. Something may happen in your life that may completely through you off track, leaving you wondering where you went wrong and debating whether or not you even have the courage to start all over again. The point is that despite all of your hard work and good intentions, obstacles are going to show up. The question is, what are you going to do about them? That means that if your program is not bringing you the results that you are after, just change it! Welcome the change, find what works for you, and enjoy yourself. I can assure you that if you stay flexible, and are willing to change whatever you need to along the way, you are on your way to creating powerful changes that will last a lifetime!

30
Go Back To The Drawing Board

Someone once said that true madness comes from doing the same things over and over again and expecting a different result. This also applies to your health and fitness program. When people become locked into certain fitness or nutrition routine, more often than not, they are going to become extremely discouraged if the routine doesn't work for them. That doesn't mean that the routine was wrong or that they weren't working hard enough. What this may be revealing is a small "glitch" in the fitness or nutrition program that may need to be addressed. In this case, their "means" may not be the most effective way for them to achieve their "end." Just remember that "failing" is not usually a question of will power, it's more often than not, a question of strategy.

The point is that you shouldn't be surprised when you have to totally regroup, completely change your program around, and start all over again. Just don't be upset because if you are just starting a new exercise or nutrition program, this is more than likely going to happen. Because in an ideal world, everything we did would work the first time, and everything we touched would turn to gold. Guess what? This isn't always the case! So start by being honest with yourself and be willing to notice whether what you are doing is working for you or not. If it is, great! If not, swallow your pride and go back to the drawing board!

31
Keep Your Momentum

Quite a few years ago, a physicist by the name of Isaac Newton made a statement that would actually apply to more areas of study than just that of his own. This one law seems to explain why there are those who, despite major adversity in their lives, have achieved such greatness, while others, despite an endless amount of opportunity at their disposal, seem to achieve so little. Newton's First Law states that an object in motion tends to stay in motion, while an object at rest tends to stay at rest. How does this law of physics apply to real life? Doesn't it seem like successful people tend to stay successful? Doesn't it also seem like people who tend to fall short of their goals seem to do so fairly consistently? Have you ever wondered why?

It should come as no surprise that success breeds even more success. Much like an athlete who seems to be in "the zone," for those people who are doing well at something, odds are that they will continue to do well, as long as they keep their momentum going. At the same time, aren't there people who always seem to be falling short of their true potential in some area of their lives? Doesn't it seem apparent that they are trapped in a downward spiral that they never seem to be able to escape from? These people become so accustomed to failing that they would have no idea how to succeed, even if they wanted to!

While there are people who seem to be "naturals" at whatever it is that they do, there are those of us who have to work extremely hard for everything that we have. As would be expected, there is a certain level of pride and appreciation that comes from working hard every single day, overcoming whatever obstacles that life presents you with, and still managing to come out on top. Once you start succeeding at anything, there are definite reasons behind it. Whatever the reasons are, be aware of what you've been doing because more often that not, you are going to be given the opportunity to see if what you did the first time has the potential of generating the same level of success in the future. Remember that success does not happen by accident, and it can be duplicated once you harness the power of momentum!

32
Believe In Yourself

We would all be extremely naïve and over–idealistic if we believed that everything we did would make everyone happy. The fact is that when it comes to taking life–changing action in any area of your lives, there are going to be those who support you, and there will be those who don't. As you progress towards achieving anything, don't be surprised if people, who you would normally expect to be extremely supportive and understanding, completely undermine what you are doing and even "bash" all of your effort and hard work. Don't listen to them! People who aren't supportive with their family and friends have usually fallen short of their own dreams and as such, they can't bear to see anyone else succeed if it doesn't involve them. In being "realistic," more often than not, people often discourage each other from pursuing what would make them happy. Could it be that misery loves company? Perhaps...

The bottom line is that despite all of your efforts to try to please the people around you, odds are that they will never be quite as happy as you would like them to be. That's when you need to dig deep and realize that no one is going to do it for you! Once you realize that you are going to have to be the sole source of inspiration, it is then when you are able to tap into the very re-source that will continue to produce explosive changes that most people only dream of.

Putting It All Together

Before we go any further, I would like to congratulate all of you for coming this far on your journey of positive lifestyle change. The fact that you've completed this book proves to me that your decision to change has already been made. You've come a long way and I hope that this book has provided some insight that can help you produce explosive changes in your own lives. Although it may seem like the book is ending, your journey has just begun. Now the time has come for you to use the tools you've learned in this book and take the first step, right now!

Throughout this book, I have done my best to inspire you to look inside to discover your reasons for creating a healthier way of life. If exercise isn't right for you, don't do it. If you completely despise "eating healthy," you don't have to do that either. My goal in writing this book was to let you know that if you do decide to change your life, I am here to help you get there. So no matter where you are now, and no matter what you decide to do with your health, I am behind each and every one of you every step of the way! Just remember that you have to know, with every ounce of conviction, that you can change your life if you want it badly enough.

Remember that life is a journey, not simply a destination. Like health and fitness, it should be enjoyed every step of the way as we constantly challenge ourselves to become the best that we can be. Whatever it is that you dream of becoming in your lives, make it happen! It is this hope for something better and something more that will continue to guide people in achieving the excellence that most people only dream of. It is this dream that has made this book a reality and I know that it can do the same for you!

I wish all of you the best of luck in your own health pursuits and all of your lifelong endeavors. Enjoy your health!

About The Author

Holding a Bachelor's degree in Nutrition and Fitness from The Florida State University, Adam has been an extremely active presenter in the field of nutrition and exercise science, health behavior modification, and peak performance consulting. As the founder of The Creative Fitness Consulting Group, he has provided nutrition counseling, health and fitness programming, and lifestyle management consulting services nationwide. Adam also speaks regularly on fitness, nutrition, stress management, as well as health and wellness program design. Adam currently lives in Chesterfield, Missouri where he is a student at Logan College of Chiropractic.

"The only way to discover the limits of the possible is to go beyond them into the impossible."

—Arthur C. Clarke